Table of Contents

Eczema is a condition that causes your skin to become dry, itchy and bumpy. This condition weakens your skin's barrier function, which is responsible for helping your skin retain moisture and protecting your body from outside elements.

Eczema is a type of dermatitis. Dermatitis is a group of conditions that cause skin inflammation.

BREAKFAST

1. Bangin Breakfast Burger

Prep Time: 5 Minutes

Cook Time: 5 Minutes

Servings: 1

Ingredients

- 1 brioche bun
- 1 egg
- ½ small avocado
- ½ small tomato
- ⅓ small red onion
- 2 green butter lettuce leaves
- 1 ½ teaspoons extra virgin olive oil
- Sprinkle of cajun seasoning
- Sea salt

Sauce:

- 1 teaspoon barbeque sauce

- 1 teaspoon whole egg mayonnaise
- 2 drops apple cider vinegar

Instructions

1. Slice onion into strips, tomato into slices and mash avocado in a small bowl.
2. Slice open burger bun and toast insides on a pan on medium heat. At the same time, mix sauce ingredients in a small bowl until combined.
3. Remove buns once toasted and sauté onions in half the olive oil.
4. Push onions to one side of the pan and crack the egg on the other side in remaining oil.
5. Season egg with cajun seasoning, sea salt and cook to your liking. I prefer the egg yolk to be runny so I don't break the yolk and cook it for approx. 3 minutes.
6. Whilst egg is cooking, spread avocado on the bottom of the burger bun, lay lettuce on top followed by the tomato. Season tomato with sea salt.
7. Add cooked onions on top of the tomato followed by the cooked egg.
8. Add sauce to the top of the burger bun and place on top to close the burger. Cut in half and dig in!

Prep Time: 5 Minutes

Cook Time: 15 Minutes

Servings: 1

Ingredients

- 1 large flour tortilla or wrap (I've used a whole grain wrap)
- 8 tater tots / potato bites
- 2 small eggs (or one large egg)
- ¼ avocado
- 3 pieces sundried tomatoes
- Sprinkle of cheddar cheese
- Hot sauce (or your favourite sauce)
- Salt and pepper

Avocado Crema:

- ½ soft avocado
- 1 heaped tbsp greek yoghurt
- ½ lime squeezed
- 2-3 tablespoon water
- Handful coriander / cilantro leaves

- Salt and pepper

Instructions

1. Make the avocado crema by adding all the ingredients to a blender and blitzing together. Start with 2-3 tablespoon of water and add slowly to achieve your preferred consistency
2. Cook the tater tots / potato bites in an air fryer or oven until they're super crispy. Approx 10 minutes at 180°C/350°F in the air fryer
3. Whisk the eggs in a bowl, then pour into a fry pan with olive oil. Over low heat, fold the eggs slowly to keep them fluffy rather than a fast scramble
4. Season with salt and pepper and take off the heat when they're almost cooked, as they continue cooking from the residual heat
5. Dice sundried tomatoes into small cubes and slice the avocado
6. Heat tortilla or wrap in the microwave for a few seconds to warm it up
7. Layer all the ingredients in the centre, neatly in a row on top of eachother. Making sure to leave room on the sides to be folded in

8. The order I've laid mine starts with the tater tots, avocado, sundried tomatoes, eggs, sauce and cheese

9. To fold the burrito, first fold the two sides over the filling, then fold the bottom half up and over the filling, tucking it in and firmly holding it together. Then continue rolling all the way up so it's a tight and compact burrito

10. Heat the burrito in a frying pan over medium heat for a few minutes turning it over so all the sides are toasted

11. Slice in half, dip into the avocado crema and enjoy your Vegetarian Breakfast Burrito!

Prep Time: 15 Minutes

Cook Time: 05 Minutes

Servings: 4

Ingredients

- 200 grams feta cheese
- 3 tablespoon greek yogurt
- 1 tablespoon extra virgin olive oil
- 1 Persian cucumber
- 1 small tomato
- Handful walnuts
- 2 radishes
- Handful fresh mint leaves
- Bread for serving - I suggest fresh crusty bread, toast, pita bread, crackers or even pita chips!

Instructions

1. Dice the cucumber and tomato into small cubes. Make sure to pat dry the tomato to remove the excess water.

Slice the radish into thin slices. Leave ingredients on the side for now

2. Crumble the block of feta cheese into smaller pieces and place in a food processor or blender. Add Greek yogurt, 2 teaspoon of olive oil and blend until smooth. Check the consistency, it should be thick and creamy. If its too clumpy, add another tablespoon of yogurt and another teaspoon of olive oil and blend again

3. Spoon the creamy whipped feta dip onto a clean large board and make swirl designs using the back of the spoon

4. Add toppings by first sprinkling the cucumbers and tomatoes, followed by the radish. Crumble over the walnuts and tear the fresh mint leaves on top

5. Lastly, garnish with a drizzle with extra virgin olive oil and serve with bread. Go for a dip with your bread or a knife and enjoy your Persian Whipped Feta "Butter" Board!

Prep Time: 20 Minutes

Cook Time: 10 Minutes

Servings: 10

Ingredients

- 500 g zucchini
- 70 g Parmigiano reggiano cheese (parmesan cheese)
- 100 g flour (I used chickpea flour)
- 1 small bunch parsley leaves (approximately 20 grams)
- 1 garlic clove
- 1 egg (to make it egg-free)
- 1 tsp baking powder
- Salt and pepper to taste
- ¼ cup oil for frying, I've used extra virgin olive oil

Instructions

1. Grate the zucchini using a box grater and place in a colander with a plate underneath. Leave aside for 10 minutes while you prepare the rest of the ingredients

2. Grate the parmigiano reggiano cheese and garlic clove
    and place in a large mixing bowl

3. Finely chop the parsley and add to the bowl with the
    egg, chickpea flour and a few pinches of salt. Stir the
    ingredients together

4. Hold the zucchini pulp in your hands and squeeze out
    the excess liquid, add to the rest of the ingredients
    and mix together

5. Heat some of the the oil in a pan on medium-high
    heat and spoon a heaped tablespoon of the batter into
    the pan. Flatten gently with the back of the spoon to
    make a circle. After a few minutes, flip and cook both
    sides until golden brown

6. Place the cooked zucchini fritters on paper towels to
    draw out the excess oil and keep continuing the prior
    step until the mixture has finished. Enjoy your
    Frittelle di Zucchine hot or cold

5. Zucchini Corn Fritters

Prep Time: 15 Minutes

Cook Time: 30 Minutes

Servings: 12

Ingredients

- 3 medium zucchini
- 1 cup corn kernels, they can be fresh/canned or frozen and thawed
- ½ red onion diced into small cubes
- 2 eggs
- ½ cup flour (I've used chickpea flour)
- 1 teaspoon baking powder
- ¼ cup parmesan cheese
- Handful of chopped coriander/cilantro or parsley
- Salt and pepper to taste
- Olive oil

Yoghurt Herb Dip:

- 5 tablespoon plain Greek yoghurt
- Good pinch of dried dill
- Salt and pepper to taste

Instructions

1. Preheat oven to 220°C /425°F and line an oven tray with baking paper
2. Place a clean tea towel in a bowl, using a box grater, grate zucchini into the towel and leave aside for 10 minutes
3. In a separate large bowl, add the corn, onion, herbs, eggs, parmesan cheese and season.
4. Now back to the shredded zucchini, hold the tea towel up, and squeeze out the excess liquid from the grated zucchini. You want to remove as much of the liquid as you can
5. Add zucchini to the other ingredients, add the flour and baking powder and mix together well.
6. Spoon some of the mixture, and using your hands, roll into balls and place on a tray lined with baking paper. If the mixture is too wet, you can add a little more flour
7. Once mixture is finished, with your fingers, gently flatten the balls slightly to resemble a round disk.
8. With a kitchen brush, brush olive oil to the tops then place tray into the oven to cook
9. After 20 minutes or when slightly golden they are done!

10. Let them rest for a few minutes on a cooling rack, stack them up and serve with a good spoon of the yoghurt dip!

11. Yoghurt Herb Dip

12. Mix yoghurt herb dip ingredients in a bowl and serve.

Prep Time: 10 Minutes

Cook Time: 0 Minutes

Servings: 1

Ingredients

- 2 Weetabix or Weet-bix
- ½ cup milk - I've used almond milk
- 1 teaspoon maple syrup or honey
- ½ banana sliced
- 100 g dairy free yogurt or Greek yoghurt

Biscoff Overnight Weetabix:

- 1 tablespoon melted biscoff spread
- 1 crushed biscoff biscuit
- Berry Overnight Weetabix
- 1-2 tsp maple syrup or honey
- Handful mixed berries

Instructions

1. Crush up the 2 Weetabix biscuits in a container or bowl. Add maple syrup or honey and milk of choice, mix together and flatten the mixture to make an even layer

2. Biscoff Overnight Weetabix

3. In a separate bowl, add the yogurt and either the melted biscoff spread and whisk together

4. Add the banana slices on top of the Weetabix layer and top with the yogurt

5. Using the back of a spoon, level out the yogurt on top

6. Place the lid on and refrigerate a few hours or overnight. To serve, top with a crushed biscoff biscuit and enjoy!

7. Berry Overnight Weetabix

8. In a separate bowl, add the yogurt a teaspoon of maple syrup/honey and whisk together

9. Using the back of a spoon, level out the yogurt on top. Then add the mixed berries on top

10. Place the lid on and refrigerate a few hours or overnight.

11. Right before serving drizzle extra honey on top and enjoy your Overnight Weetabix!

Prep Time: 5 Minutes

Cook Time: 10 Minutes

Servings: 1

Ingredients

- 2 slices whole grain sourdough bread toasted
- 1 portobello mushroom sliced
- 4 swiss brown mushrooms sliced
- 2 tablespoon ricotta cheese
- ½ small onion sliced
- 1 garlic clove diced
- 3 teaspoon olive oil
- 1 teaspoon balsamic vinegar
- Handful rocket leaves
- Salt and pepper
- Chopped parsley
- Chili flakes (optional)

Instructions

1. Sauté onion in 2 teaspoon of olive oil with a sprinkle of sea salt for a few minutes.
2. Once translucent, add garlic and sauté for a couple of minutes
3. Add mushrooms with a light drizzle of olive oil and sauté over a high heat
4. When mushrooms have browned, season with salt and pepper, add chopped parsley and remove off the heat
5. In a bowl, add rocket leaves, balsamic vinegar, light drizzle of olive oil and salt, and mix together
6. To assemble, spread ricotta cheese on toasted sourdough, add rocket leaves, layer on the sautéed mushrooms and top with a sprinkle of chili flakes and enjoy your Creamy Mushroom Toast!

Prep Time: 15 Minutes

Cook Time: 20 Minutes

Servings: 8

Ingredients

- 1 ½ cups self raising flour
- 1 cup Greek yogurt - I'm using non fat
- Pinch of salt
- Extra flour for dusting

Pizza toppings:

- ½ can Italian peeled tomatoes (or store bought pizza sauce)
- 1 teaspoon olive oil
- 10 mushrooms sliced
- 50 g kalamata olives halved
- 100 g marinated artichokes sliced
- ¼ red onion sliced
- 100 g bocconcini mozzarella halved
- 1 tablespoon basil pesto (optional)

Instructions

1. Preheat oven to 200°C/400°F
2. Add the flour, Greek yogurt and salt in a bowl and mix together with a spoon to form a ball. It's also easier to use your hands to help.
3. Transfer dough to a table or kitchen bench top. Dust with flour and knead for a few minutes until a smooth consistency is achieved. If it's too wet or sticky, sprinkle with a little more flour until it's easier to knead
4. Dust the dough with flour and using a rolling pin or bottle of wine, roll the dough to form a thin round pizza shape
5. It should be approximately 32 cm in diameter. Dust flour along the way to help roll it out
6. Carefully transfer the dough to an oven tray lined with a baking sheet
7. Add a layer of pizza sauce to the centre, leaving the outside rim for the pizza crust. Add all your toppings, except for the mozzarella and pesto
8. Put in the oven for 12 - 15 minutes until the base has browned and looks cooked
9. Add the mozzarella and put back in the oven for a further 4-5 minutes until the cheese has melted

10. Remove from oven and to serve dollop over some fresh Basil Pesto, and enjoy your easy peasy Protein Pizza!

Prep Time: 5 Minutes

Cook Time: 5 Minutes

Servings: 1

Ingredients

- ½ cup rolled oats
- ½ banana
- ½ cup almond milk
- 1 tablespoon maple syrup
- 1 teaspoon chia seeds
- ½ teaspoon baking powder
- Pinch of sea salt
- 1 square dark chocolate - 10g
- 1 tablespoon Cacao nibs
- Melted coconut oil or cooking oil spray

Instructions

1. Blend the oats in a high-speed blender to create oat flour

2. Add the milk, banana, maple syrup, baking powder and salt into the blender and blend for 10-20 seconds until well combined. It should be a thick runny cake batter-like consistency

3. Grease a small ramekin by brushing melted coconut oil or cooking spray, making sure to coat the bottom and all the sides

4. Pour the batter into the ramekin and gently tap it on the kitchen benchtop to flatten the top

5. Break the dark chocolate square into 4 pieces and place them into the centre of the ramekin. With your fingers, press them down slightly into the mixture so they are submerged

6. Sprinkle the cacao nibs on the top and place in the microwave to cook for 2 minutes. (You can also bake in the oven at 180C/360F for 20 mins)

7. Remove and check if it's cooked all the way through by sticking a toothpick into the centre. It should come out mostly clean

8. Let it cool for a few minutes then garnish by adding a drizzle of maple syrup, then dig in!

Prep Time: 5 Minutes

Cook Time: 45 Minutes

Servings: 8

Ingredients

- 1 red onion
- 2 sweet potatoes
- 2 big handfuls kale leaves
- 200 g mushrooms
- 3 garlic cloves
- 3 tablespoon olive oil
- 8 free range eggs
- 50 g feta cheese
- Salt and pepper to taste
- Olive oil spray

Instructions

1. Preheat oven to 220°C/425°F

2. Wash and dice sweet potatoes into cubes, I prefer leaving the skin on however you can also peel them. Add to a baking dish

3. Slice red onion into strips, add to the potatoes

4. Pour over ½ the oil, season with salt and pepper and add to the oven to cook for approx 20 minutes (until potatoes are cooked)

5. In the mean time, chop garlic and sauté in a pan with remaining oil over medium heat

6. Chop mushrooms, add to the garlic and once they have browned, season

7. Wash and shred kale leaves, sauté with the mushrooms

8. In a large bowl, crack the eggs, season and mix to combine

9. Add all the cooked vegetables from the oven and pan to the egg mixture, mix together quickly so the eggs don't scramble

10. Using the same oven dish, spray olive oil around the sides and bottom, pour in the egg and vegetable mixture and flatten so it's an even layer

11. Crumble over the feta cheese, add the dish to the oven and cook for 20 minutes (until the eggs are cooked).

Stick a took pick inside to check they have cooked all
the way through

12. Let the frittata cool for 5-10 minutes, slice into pieces
and enjoy!

11. Tahini Kale Salad with Crispy Chickpeas

Prep Time: 10 Minutes

Cook Time: 20 Minutes

Servings: 5

Ingredients

- 600 g sweet potatoes
- 1 can chickpeas
- 2-3 tablespoon olive oil
- 1 ½ teaspoon smoked paprika
- 1 teaspoon garlic powder
- 160 g kale leaves2 Persian or Lebanese cucumbers
- Salt and pepper

Dressing:

- ⅓ cup tahini
- 1 ½ lemons
- 3-4 tablespoon cold water
- Salt

Garnish:

- Pickled onions

Instructions

1. Preheat oven to 200°C/400°F
2. Dice sweet potatoes into small bite sized cubes and place on one side of a baking tray
3. Drain a can of chickpeas, dry them and place on the other side of the baking tray
4. Season all with olive oil, salt and pepper. Season the chickpeas with paprika and garlic powder and mix with your hands
5. Bake in the oven for 20 - 25 minutes until golden and crispy. Tip, leave only chickpeas in the oven for an extra 5-10 minutes with the temperature off to get them super crispy. Here are more tips
6. To make the dressing, add tahini, lemon juice and salt to a small bowl. Start with 3 tablespoons of cold water and whisk together well until its runny but still creamy. If it seems too thick, add another tablespoon of water. Always start with less as you can keep adding more if needed

7. Chop the kale leaves very finely and place in a large salad bowl. Add tablespoon of olive oil and massage the oil with your hands into the kale leaves

8. Add the cooked sweet potatoes and diced cucumbers to the salad bowl. Pour over the dressing and toss it well together so everything is nicely coated.

9. Top with the crispy chickpeas, garnish with pickled onions and its ready to be eaten as a main or side dish!

Prep Time: 10 Minutes

Cook Time: 5 Minutes

Servings: 20

Ingredients

- 1 baguette
- 10 cherry tomatoes
- 1-2 Persian or Lebanese cucumbers
- 150 g olive spread
- 100 g feta cheese
- ¼ red onion
- Drizzle of olive oil
- Garlic clove

Dressing:

- 3 tablespoon extra virgin olive oil
- 1 tablespoon white vinegar
- ½ lemon
- 1 teaspoon dried oregano
- Pinch of Salt

Instructions

1. Prepare veggies by slicing the cherry tomatoes into half and slicing the onion thinly. Using a peeler, peel the cucumber to make cucumber ribbons

2. Add all dressing ingredients to a small bowl or ramekin and whisk together

3. Slice the baguette diagonally into about 20 slices. Lay flat on a tray with a baking sheet and drizzle lightly with olive oil. Put in a pre-heated oven at 180°C/350°F for 3-4 minutes until nicely toasted.

4. Remove from oven and rub the toasted baguette slices with the garlic clove

5. Assemble by spreading on the olive spread, top with a rolled cucumber ribbon, half a cherry tomatoand a couple red onion slices. Crumble over the feta, drizzle over some dressing and they're ready to be served!

Prep Time: 5 Minutes

Cook Time: 25 Minutes

Servings: 6

Ingredients

- 6 medium portobello mushrooms
- 150 g frozen spinach thawed
- 130 g ricotta cheese
- 50 g sundried tomatoes
- Sea salt
- Olive oil spary

Crumb:

- 15 g panko breadcrumbs
- 10 g freshly grated parmigiano reggiano cheese
- Garlic powder
- Extra virgin olive oil

Instructions

1. Preheat oven to 220°C/425°F

2. Cut the stems off the mushrooms and wipe the outides clean with damp power towels (don't throw away stems as you can use them in a future dish)

3. Place mushrooms facing down on an oven tray, preferably on a wire rack. This is so extra moisture can drip off the mushrooms into the tray. Cook in the oven for 10-15 minutes (until cooked)

4. In the mean time, drain and press the excess liquid from the spinach with a small colander and add to a bowl.

5. Add ricotta to the bowl, season with sea salt and mix together

6. In a separate bowl, make the crumb by adding panko breadcrumbs, parmigiano reggiano, with a sprinkle of garlic powder and drizzle of olive oil

7. When mushrooms are cooked, remove from the oven and pat dry

8. Fill each mushroom evenly with the mixture

9. Add sundried tomatoes on top of each mushroom, you can also chop into smaller strips if they are whole or large

10. Sprinkle each mushroom with the crumb and place back into the oven for 10 minutes

11. If crumb hasn't browned enough, you can place under the grill for a few minutes, just keep an eye on them as the crumb can burn quickly

12. Serve and enjoy as either an appetizer or main meal!

Prep Time: 10 Minutes

Cook Time: 25 Minutes

Servings: 6

Ingredients

- 1 tablespoon olive oil
- 1 large onion chopped
- 2 garlic cloves minced
- 2-3 large carrots chopped
- 2-3 celery stalks chopped
- 6 cups vegetable broth
- 1 teaspoon dried thyme
- ½ teaspoon oregano
- 1 teaspoon salt
- ½ teaspoon black pepper
- 3 15-ounces canned white beans drained and rinsed
- 2 cups baby spinach
- Fresh parsley finely chopped, for serving
- Grated parmesan cheese for serving

Instructions

1. In a large pot or saucepan, heat olive over medium high heat. Add onions and cook until onions are translucent, about 3-5 minutes. Add the garlic, carrots, celery, thyme, oregano, salt and pepper, and cook for an additional 2-3 minutes.
2. Add vegetable broth and beans, bring to a boil, reduce heat and simmer for 15 minutes to combine all of the flavors together.
3. Stir in the spinach and continue to simmer until the spinach wilts, about 2 minutes
4. Remove from heat, sprinkle fresh parsley and grated parmesan cheese, if desired, and serve immediately.

Prep Time: 10 Minutes

Cook Time: 30 Minutes

Servings: 6

Ingredients

- 3 tablespoons extra-virgin olive oil
- 1 medium onion diced
- 2 celery stalks sliced
- 2 large carrots sliced
- Salt and pepper to taste
- 4 yukon potatoes diced (3-4 cups chopped)
- 1 teaspoon dried thyme
- 2 garlic cloves minced
- 3 cups low-sodium vegetable broth
- 2 cups peas frozen
- 2 cups corn frozen
- 2 cups plant-based milk
- Fresh parsley for serving

Instructions

1. Heat the olive oil in a large pot over medium heat. Add the onions, celery and carrots to the pot. Season with salt and pepper. Cook, stirring occasionally until vegetables start to soften, about 5 minutes.

2. Stir in the chopped potatoes, thyme and garlic and cook until fragrant, about 1 minute. Add the vegetable broth. Bring mixture to a boil, then simmer until the vegetables soften, about 20 minutes.

3. Use an immersion blender to lightly blend the soup so it's thicker but still chunky. You can remove some of the vegetables aside to stir back in if you prefer to have more whole vegetables.

4. Stir in the peas, corn and milk, and simmer until the vegetables are warmed through and soup has thickened, about 5 minutes.

5. Serve with fresh parsley and crusty bread, if desired.

Prep Time: 5 Minutes

Cook Time: 20 Minutes

Servings: 2

Ingredients

- 1 zucchini sliced
- 1 yellow squash sliced
- 1 eggplant sliced
- 1 red pepper sliced
- ¼ cup red onions sliced
- Olive oil spray
- ½ teaspoon dill
- Salt and pepper to taste
- 2 tablespoons butter
- 4 slices thick bread
- 4 ounces Dill Havarti cheese divided
- 4 ounces Gouda cheese divided

Instructions

1. Preheat oven to 400°F. Toss the vegetables with olive oil spray and dill and season with salt and pepper. Spread out on a baking sheet and roast for 10 minutes, until vegetables are slightly tender.
2. Brush the melted butter on one side of the bread slices.
3. In a large cast iron skillet or electric griddle over medium low heat, place one slice of bread on the skillet, buttered side down. Add half the Dill Havarti cheese on top of the bread, then layer with half the roasted vegetables, followed by half the Gouda cheese. Top with a bread slice, buttered side up.
4. Cook grilled cheese sandwich until golden brown and cheese is melted, about 4-6 minutes on each side. Repeat for the second sandwich.

Prep Time: 10 Minutes

Cook Time: 10 Minutes

Servings: 8

Ingredients

- 500 g short pasta (I've used Fusilli)
- 500 g cherry tomatoes
- 180 g kalamata pitted olives
- 1 red onion
- 2 bunches parsley leaves chopped finely
- 50 g feta cheese

Dressing:

- 1 lemon squeezed
- ⅓ cup extra virgin olive oil
- Salt and pepper to taste

Instructions

1. Dice onion into small cubes

2. Slice cherry tomatoes along with kalamata olives into halves.

3. Boil pasta to al dente in heavily salted water (refer to instructions on packet for the timing). Note don't overcook the pasta as it will become mushy.

4. While the pasta is cooking, pour dressing ingredients into a large bowl and whisk until combined. Reemember not to add too much salt as the olives and feta are quite salty.

5. Add half of the chopped parsley to the dressing

6. Once pasta is cooked, strain and add straight to the big bowl with the dressing while its still hot. Mix well so the dressing coats all the pasta.

7. Let stand for 5-10 minutes until it has cooled, then add all ingredients except for the feta. Mix until all well combined.

8. Crumble over the feta upon serving alongside your favourite protein or enjoy on it's own. This salad also works great as a side dish for a barbeque or picnic salad

Prep Time: 8 Minutes

Cook Time: 5 Minutes

Servings: 2

Ingredients

- 1 Persian/ Lebanese cucumber
- 5 cherry tomatoes
- ¼ bell pepper/ capsicum
- ¼ small red onion
- 30 g kalamata olives
- 30 g feta cheese
- 60 g chickpeas
- 4 tablespoon tzatziki
- 2 romaine lettuce leaves
- 2 wraps or tortillas

Dressing:

- 2 tablespoon extra virgin olive oil
- 2 tablespoon vinegar (I've used white wine vinegar)
- 1 teaspoon oregano
- ½ garlic clove

- Pinch of salt

Instructions

1. Dice the cucumber, tomatoes, capsicum, onion and olives into cubes and add to a large bowl
2. Add the chickpeas and crumble over the feta cheese
3. Add the dressing ingredients to a small bowl or jar and stir together. Pour over the salad and mix together
4. Assemble the wrap by spreading the tzatziki sauce to the middle of the wrap lengthways. Place the romaine lettuce on top of the tzatziki in a strip and spoon half of the greek salad mixture into the lettuce leaf
5. Fold the top and bottom of the wrap in, then roll the wrap lengthways like a burrito. Slice in half and enjoy your Greek wrap!

20. Unagi (Japanese Eel) Sushi Roll

Prep Time: 15 Minutes

Cook Time: 15 Minutes

Servings: 4

Ingredients

For Sushi Rice:

- 1.5 tablespoons sugar
- 1 teaspoon salt
- 1.5 tablespoons apple cider vinegar
- 1.5 tablespoons rice vinegar
- 3 cups cooked short-grain rice (You can use white or brown)
- For Unagi Roll:
- 4 seaweed/nori sheets
- 1 cooked unagi
- 1 English cucumber, cut into thin match sticks
- ½ avocado, cut into strips
- ½ red bell pepper, cut into thin strips
- Wasabi and soy sauce for serving

Instructions

1. Cook unagi according to the package. I like to cook mine in the toaster oven and broil it at the end for a couple of minutes. Broiling caramelizes the sauce and yields a better texture for the unagi.

2. While you are cooking unagi, prepare your sushi rice. In a small bowl, mix together sugar, salt, and vinegar until sugar and salt dissolve completely. Use half of this mixture over cooked rice and mix. Taste the rice and adjust the seasoning to your liking. Let the rice cool to room temperature. Make sure to cover your rice with a kitchen towel so the rice won't dry up.

3. Once the unagi is cooked, cut into strips length-wise. Set them aside.

4. Prepare the vegetable. Cut the cucumber and red bell pepper into thin match sticks and cut the avocado into thick strips. Set them aside.

5. Assemble unagi roll. On a piece of nori/seaweed paper, evenly spread ¼ of the seasoned sushi rice. If the sushi rice is sticking to your hand, wet your hand with water and use your fingertips to spread the rice. Place the cooked unagi, cucumber, red bell pepper, and avocado on top of the rice. Grab the bottom of the seaweed paper and place it over so it covers the

fillings. Carefully roll the roll and give it a gentle squeeze.

6. Once you are done rolling the roll, place the roll on the dish, seam side down. Repeat until all rolls are assembled.

7. When ready to serve the roll, wet your knife with water and slice the roll in sawing motion. Wetting your knife prevents sushi rice to stick to the knife. You can serve the rolls with wasabi and soy sauce.

21. Bok Choy Mushroom Pasta Stir Fry

Prep Time: 5 Minutes

Cook Time: 20 Minutes

Servings: 3

Ingredients

- 7 to 8 ounces pasta of your choice
- 1 tablespoon low sodium soy sauce
- 1 tablespoon dark soy sauce
- 1 tablespoon vegetarian oyster sauce
- 1 tablespoon pasta water
- ½ tablespoon maple syrup
- 1 tablespoon oil
- 2 cloves of garlic, minced (1 to 2 teaspoons of minced garlic)
- 3 cups bok choy, roughly chopped
- 1 package mushroom, sliced

Instructions

1. Cook the pasta according to its package. Reserve a tablespoon of pasta cooking water.

2. While the pasta is cooking, mix together low-sodium soy sauce, dark soy sauce, vegetarian oyster sauce, maple syrup, and pasta cooking water. Set aside.

3. Prepare your vegetables (roughly chop bok choy and slice the mushrooms).

4. In a non-stick skillet, add the oil and minced garlic. Cook the minced garlic for 45 seconds until fragrant.

5. Add the mushroom to the pan. The mushroom seems to absorb all the boil but as it cooks, it will release water. Cook for 2 minutes and stir occasionally. Once the mushroom release water and soften, add the chopped bok choy.

6. Stir frequently and continue to cook until bok choy is wilted for about 3 minutes.

7. Add the cooked pasta and pour the prepared sauce. Stir to mix until everything is well coated with the sauce.

8. After 3 to 4 minutes of cooking, turn off the heat and serve.

Prep Time: 10 Minutes

Cook Time: 10 Minutes

Servings: 6

Ingredients

- 6 sweet dinner roll, cut in half
- 4 tablespoons pesto of your choice
- 1 to 2 fresh mozzarella cheese balls, sliced
- 2 small tomatoes, sliced
- Salt and pepper to taste
- Red pepper flakes (optional)
- 2 to 3 tablespoons balsamic glaze

Instructions

1. Place the sliced mozzarella cheese on a clean kitchen towel or paper towel to absorb its access water.
2. Slice the dinner roll in half. Slice the tomato and set it aside.
3. Spread 1 teaspoon of pesto on the bottom of each roll.

4. Spread 1 teaspoon of pesto on the top part of each roll. Set them aside.

5. Place the sliced mozzarella cheese and tomato on the bottom of each roll.

6. Sprinkle with salt, pepper, and red pepper flakes.

7. Drizzle with balsamic glaze.

8. Top with the other half of the roll and serve right away.

Prep Time: 10 Minutes

Cook Time: 20 Minutes

Servings: 4

Ingredients

- 1 package of vegan sausage of your choice (I use Beyond sausage Brat flavor)
- 1 tablespoon vegetable oil
- ½ cup chopped celery (2 to 3 stalks)
- 1 cup diced onion
- 3 cloves of garlic, minced
- 1 cup diced bell pepper
- 1 can diced tomato (14.5 oz)
- 2 teaspoons sugar
- 1 tablespoon creole seasoning
- 1 teaspoon dried oregano
- Black pepper to taste
- Cooked rice, short-grain pasta, mashed potato, or polenta (for serving)

Instructions

1. On a large skillet, cook the vegan sausage according to its package. If you are using Beyond sausage, there is no need to add the oil. As the sausage cooks, it releases oil from the sausage.

2. Once the sauce is cooked, take them out and slice them into bite-size pieces. Return the sausage to the pan and brown the sausage pieces for a couple of minutes.

3. Take the sausage out of the pan and set them aside.

4. On the same skillet, add 1 tablespoon of oil, celery, and onion. Cook them until the onion becomes translucent.

5. Add the minced garlic and cook with frequent stirring for 30 to 45 seconds until you smell the garlic cooking.

6. Add the bell pepper to the mixture. Cook for a minute or two.

7. Add the diced tomato, sugar, Creole seasoning, oregano, and black pepper to the mixtures.

8. Bring the sauce to a boil. Once it comes to a boil, reduce the heat to simmer, put the cooked sausage back into the skillet. Stir to mix and place a lid. Cook for an additional 10 to 15 minutes.

9. Serve over cooked rice.

Prep Time: 10 Minutes

Cook Time: 15 Minutes

Servings: 4

Ingredients

- 1 box of red lentil pasta, cooked according to its package
- 2 tablespoons sun-dried tomato in olive oil
- 2 cloves of garlic, minced
- ¼ large onion, diced
- 1 large bell pepper, diced
- 1 small size zucchini, diced
- 1 cup cherry tomato
- ½ teaspoon dried basil
- ⅓ cup raw cashew
- 1 cup hot water
- 1 tablespoon tomato paste
- ½ cup to 1 cup vegetable broth
- Salt and pepper to taste

Instructions

1. Cook the red lentil pasta according to its package.

2. Meanwhile, start cooking the minced garlic with sun-dried tomato in olive oil in the skillet. When the garlic starts to smell fragrant, add the onion, bell pepper, zucchini, cherry tomato, and dried basil. Cook for 5 minutes with frequent stirring.

3. In a high-speed blender, blend raw cashew, hot water, and tomato paste until smooth.

4. Add the cashew tomato cream sauce to the mixture in the pan. Stir to mix everything together.

5. Add the cooked pasta to the sauce

6. Add the vegetable broth until it reaches the consistency you desire.

7. Season with salt and pepper.

Prep Time: 15 Minutes

Cook Time: 25 Minutes

Servings: 4

Ingredients

- ½ zucchini
- ½ yellow squash
- ½ teaspoon salt + more to taste
- 1 tablespoon olive oil
- ½ cup chopped onion
- ½ cup chopped bell pepper
- 1 small size roman tomato, chopped
- 1 teaspoon cumin
- ½ teaspoon chili powder
- ¼ teaspoon pepper
- 1 can black bean, drained and rinsed
- ¾ cup Mexican blend cheese (or cheese of your choice)
- 1 and ½ cup of red enchilada sauce
- 5 to 6 tortillas (I use 10-inch flour tortillas)
- Avocado, jalapeno, and/or queso fresco (for garnish)

Instructions

1. Wash the zucchini and yellow squash and them in half, lengthwise. Cut the zucchini and yellow squash in half lengthwise again and cut out the seeds. Cut them once more by half, lengthwise. Dice the zucchini and yellow squash into small cube pieces.

2. In a shallow bowl, place a clean paper towel on the bottom and transfer the cut zucchini and yellow squash on top. Sprinkle about ½ teaspoon of salt over them. Gently toss together so the salt can cover the zucchini and yellow squash evenly. Let them salt while you prepare other vegetables.

3. Heat a tablespoon of oil in a large skillet. Add the onion and bell pepper. Cook until onion becomes translucent, about 3-4 minutes.

4. Add the chopped tomato to the mixture and continue to cook for couple more minutes.

5. Using the paper towel, pat the zucchini and yellow squash dry. Add the zucchini and yellow squash to the mixture.

6. Add the black bean, cumin, chili powder, and black pepper to the mixture and stir until everything is well mixed. Add about a pinch of salt to the mixture.

7. Remove the mixture from heat.

8. Add about ⅔ cup of red enchilada sauce and ½ cup of cheese to the vegetable mixture. Mix well.

9. Preheat the oven to 400F.

10. While the oven is preheating, assemble the enchiladas.

11. Place about ½ cup of red enchilada sauce on the bottom of a 9 x 9 inches baking pan. Spread the sauce so the bottom is completely covered with the sauce.

12. Place about ½ cup of the vegetable mixture on top of tortillas and roll them tightly. Transfer to the baking dish, the seam side down. Repeat until all the vegetable mixture is used up.

13. Pour the rest of the enchilada sauce on top of the assembled enchiladas and sprinkle with the rest of the cheese.

14. Bake for 16-18 minutes. Garnish with fresh avocado, jalapeno slices, and/or queso fresco. Serve right away.

Prep Time: 25 Minutes

Cook Time: 25 Minutes

Servings: 2

Ingredients

Sushi Rice

- 3 cups cooked sushi rice (short grain rice)
- 1 tablespoon apple cider vinegar
- 1 tablespoon rice wine vinegar
- 1 tablespoon sugar
- ½ teaspoon salt

Spicy Mayo Sauce:

- 3 tablespoons vegan mayo
- 1 tablespoon sweet chili sauce
- 1 tablespoon sriracha

Sushi Bowl:

- 4 to 6 vegan fishless filets, cooked according to package (I used Gardein's Golden Fishless Filet)
- ⅓ English cucumber, diced into small cubes

- 2 small avocados or 1 large avocado, diced
- 1 small green onion, thinly sliced (for garnish)

Instructions

1. Bake the vegan fishless filets according to their package.
2. While the fishless filets are baking, mix together apple cider vinegar, rice wine vinegar, sugar, and salt in a small bowl. Stir until sugar and salt are dissolved. Add the mixture to the cooked sushi rice. Set aside.
3. In another small bowl, mix together vegan mayo, sweet chili sauce, and sriracha. Set aside.
4. Assemble the sushi bowl. Place the seasoned sushi rice in a bowl, about 1 and ½ cups. Add the diced cucumber, vegan fishless filets, and avocado. Drizzle with vegan spicy mayo sauce. Garnish with green onion.

Prep Time: 10 Minutes

Cook Time: 15 Minutes

Servings: 2

Ingredients

- 2 tablespoons vegetarian stir fry sauce (vegetarian oyster sauce)
- 2 tablespoons soy sauce
- 1 tablespoon chili garlic sauce (sambal oelek)
- 3 tablespoons grapeseed oil (or vegetable oil)
- 6 to 8 cloves garlic, minced
- 1 cup chopped bell pepper
- 1-2 jalapeños chopped (seeds removed before chopping)
- 3 bird's eye chili (optional)
- 4 cups cooked rice (jasmine rice or short-grain sushi rice)
- Sriracha sauce (for serving, optional)

Instructions

1. In a small bowl, mix together vegetarian stir fry sauce (vegetarian oyster sauce), soy sauce, and chili garlic sauce. Set aside.

2. Prepare your vegetable. Mince the garlic and finely dice the bell pepper. Remove the seeds and membrane of the jalapeño and dice finely. If you are using bird's eye chili, only use the bottom half of the peppers.

3. Place the prepared sauce and vegetables near the stove so you can add them quickly.

4. On a large non-stick skillet, heat about 3 tablespoons of oil. Add the minced garlic and cook until they turn slightly brown.

5. As soon as the garlic turns light brown, add the diced jalapeño, bell pepper, and bird's eye chili. Fry them with frequent stirring for a couple of minutes.

6. Add the rice to the mixture and pour the sauce over the rice.

7. Continue to fry and mix until everything is well incorporated.

8. Serve with extra chili garlic sauce or sriracha sauce.

Prep Time: 5 Minutes

Cook Time: 15 Minutes

Servings: 2

Ingredients

- 2 cups sliced bell pepper and onion
- ½ tablespoon olive oil
- ¼ teaspoon salt
- Pinch of freshly ground black pepper
- 1.5 lb of pizza dough of your choice (or half of this recipe (using a stand mixer) or this recipe (by hand)), divide in half
- 6 to 8 provolone cheese slices
- 2 links Vegan Italian Sausage, cooked and sliced (for a vegetarian option - I used beyond sausage Hot Italian)
- 2 links sausage of your choice, cooked and sliced
- 1 cup shredded mozzarella cheese
- Dash of red pepper flakes (optional)

Instructions

1. Preheat the oven to 450F.

2. In a large size non-stick skillet, heat the olive oil to the pan and cook the peppers and onions. Once the onion turns slightly transparent but still crisp (about 3-4 minutes), turn the heat off and season with salt and pepper.

3. On a baking sheet, place the pizza dough (I made one medium size vegetarian pizza and one regular sausage and pepper pizza).

4. Add the provolone cheese on top of the pizza dough.

5. Add the cooked peppers and onions, cooked sausage, and mozzarella cheese. Sprinkle the pizza with red pepper flakes for heat (optional).

6. Bake in the oven for 10 to 12 minutes until all the cheese melts. Serve right away.

Prep Time: 10 Minutes

Cook Time: 15 Minutes

Servings: 4

Ingredients

- ¼ cup raw cashew
- ½ cup unsweetened almond milk
- 1 tablespoon oil
- 1 tablespoon vegan butter (or use another tablespoon of oil)
- ½ large onion, diced
- 2 teaspoons ginger, minced or grated
- 3 cloves garlic, minced
- 1 teaspoon cumin
- 1 teaspoon garam masala (I like this brand)
- ½ tablespoon curry powder
- ¼ teaspoon turmeric powder
- ½ teaspoon paprika
- ¼ teaspoon ground black pepper
- 3 tablespoons tomato paste
- 1 cup cauliflower floret

- 1 cup diced potato
- 2-3 small size carrots, cut into small pieces
- ½ teaspoon salt
- 1 cup water (or vegetable broth)
- 2 teaspoons Vegan Chicken Flavor Bouillon Powder (omit if using vegetable broth)
- ½ cup frozen peas
- Rice and/or naan for serving

Instructions

1. In a high-speed blender, blend together cashew and almond milk until smooth. Set aside.
2. In a large non-stick skillet, heat oil and butter together and add diced onion. Cook until onion becomes translucent.
3. Add the minced garlic and ginger. Cook until fragrant, about a minute.
4. Add tomato paste, cumin, garam masala, curry powder, turmeric, paprika, and black pepper. Stir until everything is well mixed and bubbles a little in the pan.

5. Add cauliflower carrot, potato, water, and vegan chicken flavor bouillon powder (or vegetable broth). Add the salt.

6. Bring the mixture to a boil and place a lid on top. Reduce the heat to medium and continue to cook for 5-7 minutes until the potato is cooked but not mushy.

7. Add the cashew almond milk mixture and frozen pea to the curry. Stir to mix and continue to cook for additional 2-3 minutes.

8. Serve hot with rice and/or naan.

Prep Time: 5 Minutes

Cook Time: 15 Minutes

Servings: 2

Ingredients

For the sauce:

- 2 tablespoons low-sodium soy sauce
- 1 tablespoon sweet soy sauce
- 1 tablespoon brown sugar
- ½ tablespoon garlic chili sauce

For Fried Rice:

- 2 cups cooked rice, at least a day old
- 2 tablespoons vegetable oil
- 5-7 cloves garlic, minced
- 2 red Thai peppers, minced (optional)
- ½ large onion, diced
- ½ cup bell pepper, diced
- 1 cup loosely packed fresh Thai basil

Instructions

1. In a small bowl, mix everything for the sauce and set it aside.

2. Prepare all of your vegetables. I dice my bell pepper first, then onion, and red Thai pepper/chili. I also rinse the Thai basil in cold water and dry it with a paper towel. Pick the leaves and tear them into bite sizes if the leaves are too big.

3. In a large non-stick pan, add 2 tablespoons of vegetable oil. Add minced garlic and Thai red pepper/chili. Cook with frequent stirring until the garlic turns to light brown color. If you are adding Thai pepper, it will smell smoky and spicy. It may make you cough, but we are adding a lot of ingredients that will balance the spiciness.

4. Add chopped onion and bell pepper. Cook for a minute or two with frequent stirring.

5. Add the rice and pour the sauce on top. Stir until everything is well mixed.

6. Turn off the heat and remove the pan from the heat and add the Thai basil. Mix one last time until the Thai basil is slightly wilted and mixed into the rice.